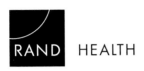

RAND HEALTH

The Role of Health Care Transformation for the Chinese Dream

Powering Economic Growth, Promoting a Harmonious Society

Soeren Mattke, Hangsheng Liu, Lauren E. Hunter,

Kun Gu, Sydne Newberry

T0306453

The research in this report was produced within RAND Health, a unit of the RAND Corporation. The research was funded by Aetna, Inc.

Library of Congress Cataloging-in-Publication Data is available for this publication.

ISBN: 978-0-8330-8566-5

The RAND Corporation is a nonprofit institution that helps improve policy and decisionmaking through research and analysis. RAND's publications do not necessarily reflect the opinions of its research clients and sponsors.

Support RAND—make a tax-deductible charitable contribution at www.rand.org/giving/contribute.html

RAND® is a registered trademark.

RAND OFFICES
SANTA MONICA, CA • WASHINGTON, DC
PITTSBURGH, PA • NEW ORLEANS, LA • JACKSON, MS • BOSTON, MA
CAMBRIDGE, UK • BRUSSELS, BE
www.rand.org

Preface

After having successfully expanded health insurance coverage, China now faces the challenge of building an effective and efficient delivery system to serve its large and aging population. The country must choose whether to follow the models of Western countries, which have well-known limitations, or create an innovative and sustainable model. In this report, we argue that China should choose the second option and design and implement a health care system based on population health management principles and sophisticated health information technology. Taking this path could yield a triple dividend for China: Health care will contribute to the growth of service sector employment, stimulate domestic demand by unlocking savings, and enable China to export its health system development capabilities to other countries, mirroring its success in building other critical infrastructure. These forces can help turn the Chinese Dream into a reality.

This research was conducted under contract with Aetna, Inc. The authors would like to express their gratitude to Drs. Jack Chow, Yuanli Liu, and Getu Zhaori for providing their insights to this report.

This research was conducted by RAND Health Advisory Services, the consulting practice of of RAND Health. A profile of RAND Health, abstracts of its publications, and ordering information can be found at www.rand.org/health. Comments or inquiries concerning this report should be sent to the lead author, Soeren Mattke, at Soeren_Mattke@rand.org or to his address at RAND: RAND Corporation, 20 Park Plaza, Suite 920, Boston, MA 02116, phone +1 (617) 338 2059.

Contents

Figures

Summary

After having successfully expanded health insurance coverage, China now faces the challenge of building an effective and efficient delivery system to serve its large and aging population. The country finds itself at a crossroads—it can emulate the models of Western countries with their well-known limitations, or embark on an ambitious endeavor to create an innovative and sustainable model. In this report, we argue that China should choose the second option and design and implement a health care system based on population health management (PHM) principles and sophisticated health information technology (IT). Taking this path can yield a triple dividend for China: Health care will contribute to the growth of service sector employment, stimulate domestic demand by unlocking savings, and enable China to export its health system development capabilities to other countries, mirroring its success in building other critical infrastructure. These forces can help turn the Chinese Dream into a reality.

China's Economic Progress Is Outpacing Its Health Care System

Since 1980, China has experienced breathtaking economic growth: Its Gross Domestic Product has grown by an average of 10 percent annually and its economy is currently the second largest in the world. With this economic boom has come a precipitous fall in the poverty rate, an equally steep rise in the standard of living, and a nearly 75-percent increase in life expectancy. However, the rapid industrialization of the country has resulted in urbanization and lifestyle changes, such as decline in physical activity, increased preference for Western diets, and a smoking rate that is nearly twice the world average, according to data from the Organization for Economic Cooperation and Development. Combined with population aging, these changes have resulted in what health researchers are calling the epidemiological transition from acute to chronic disease, resulting in a higher burden of disease and disability that has not yet been matched by increased health system capacity. To address this mismatch, China will need to repeat its success in achieving high standards in maternal and child health and improving care for acute illness. But reaching similar standards in chronic care will require a transformational approach rather than an incremental one. The growth in chronic disease prevalence is on a path to overwhelm the health care system in its current form, with its reliance on hospital care and physician services. Without such transformation, China will face a sicker population, threatening not only its vision for a harmonious society, but also its economic development.

The Economic Opportunity in Health Care Transformation

In this report, we argue that rapid economic and societal development provides China a unique opportunity to design and implement a health care system that meets the needs of the 21st century—one that is built on evidence and operated with industrial principles of process optimization and the use of advanced IT. China occupies a unique position, even among large modernizing countries, in having the opportunity to build such a world-class health care system from the ground up. Legacy infrastructure and entrenched interests are holding back health care transformation in Western countries; China is less encumbered by these and can adapt an innovative model for health care delivery that is purposefully designed for the 21st century, rather than emulating inefficient models that exist elsewhere. This novel type of health care system could avoid past mistakes and enable China to focus on what has been referred to as the three-part aim: better care, better health, and lower cost.

Transforming health care has the potential to support broader economic growth in a sustainable fashion and, importantly, to enable China's transition from an economy centered on labor and natural resources to one that is knowledge-based, as is called for in the current five-year plan. In developed countries, health care is one of the largest segments of the service sector, accounting for 7 to 16 percent of the economy, and a substantial contributor to the creation of qualified jobs. In addition, access to high-quality and affordable health care can stimulate domestic consumption by unlocking household savings set aside for health care expenditures.

Population Health Management as the Pioneering Model for World-Class Health Care

We would argue that China's future health care system should follow two design principles. First, to cope with the relative shortage of health care professionals, it needs to leverage highly skilled workers through sophisticated health IT and by shifting tasks to less-trained workers. Second, China should adopt a PHM model, which unites the public health perspective of improving health at the population level and the medical care perspective of individual care delivery.

The PHM model is characterized by three key principles: a focus on the health outcomes of the entire population; coordination of health and medical services through the continuum of care needs, from prevention and health promotion to curative care, disease management, and palliative care; and proactive management of care needs. PHM addresses health care needs from health and wellness to coping with the end of life and encompasses all dimensions of health, including physical, mental, and social well-being (Figure S.1).

Figure S.1
Health Needs Across the Continuum of Care

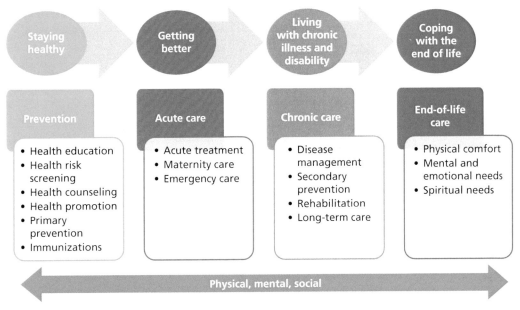

Our proposed PHM blueprint for China's future health care systems has six inter-related components (Figure S.2):

Figure S.2
The Interdependent Components of the PHM Model

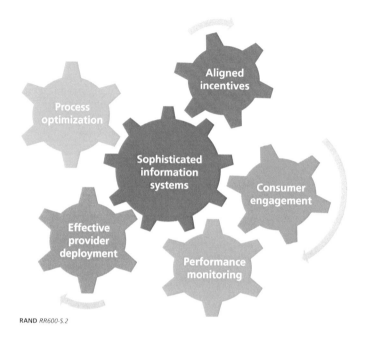

RAND *RR600-S.2*

- **A sophisticated IT infrastructure** will serve as the central cog for the model, as its data and decision support will drive the other components.
- **Data-driven optimization of care processes** will allow evidence-based care delivery and will perform gap analysis to identify future research needs.
- **Performance monitoring at all levels of accountability** will permit benchmarking, investigation of root causes for underperformance and remediation, and identification of best and worst performers to identify best practices.
- **Effective deployment of health professionals** will maximize the productivity of highly skilled professionals by task-shifting, allowing paraprofessionals to perform tasks requiring less skill and training while the country begins to develop the needed health care workforce. Assisting effective deployment will be care team formation, using a model featuring health navigators, specialized paraprofessionals who guide patients through the system.
- **Alignment of incentives with policy goals**—namely, better health processes and outcomes and lower cost—will require several considerations. Payment cannot be

tied to care settings, but must follow patients. The payment system must be based on value, not volume.

- **Consumer engagement** means patients must have some accountability for their care: They must be informed of their choices as well as the consequences of those choices.

Conclusion

China's economic and social progress over the past 30 years has outpaced its health care system. The health of China's population is being influenced simultaneously by a rapid rate of aging, growing wealth, and migration from rural to urban living, as well as an increasing reliance on food of low nutritional value and decreasing physical activity. The result is an expanding burden of chronic disease and disability, even as mortality due to acute illness wanes. To handle the new challenges, the Chinese health care system must undergo a transformation.

The current health care system is handicapped by workforce shortages, overreliance on hospital-based care, and a lack of robust IT. Although the central government is investing substantial resources, the system cannot expand quickly enough to meet expected demand, at least not with traditional delivery models. But China has the unique opportunity to chart a different course and adapt an innovative model for health care delivery that is purposefully designed for the 21st century, rather than emulating inefficient models that exist elsewhere.

This PHM model will focus on the needs of citizens and patients and will offer continuous support at all stages of health. It will make use of sophisticated IT to leverage scarce medical professionals, improve quality, promote evidence-based care and accountability, and facilitate planning. The model will also provide a source of service-sector jobs, not just in care delivery and management, but also in IT, and will help to promote economic growth by unlocking domestic savings. Thus, visionary leaders who embark on this ambitious agenda to transform health care in China can divert discontent about access to quality care as a threat to social harmony and use health care to promote the realization of the Chinese Dream.

Abbreviations

ACO	accountable care organization
BMI	body mass index
BQS	Federal Office for Quality Assurance (Germany)
COPD	chronic obstructive pulmonary disease
CPC	Communist Party of China
EHR	electronic health record
GDP	gross domestic product
GP	general practitioner
IT	information technology
NCMS	New Cooperative Medical Scheme
NCD	noncommunicable disease
OECD	Organization for Economic Cooperation and Development
PHM	population health management
UEBMI	Urban Employee Basic Medical Insurance
URBMI	Urban Resident Basic Medical Insurance

CHAPTER ONE

The Policy Argument for Rethinking Health Care in China

After three decades of breathtaking economic growth in which its gross domestic product (GDP) grew by 10 percent annually (World Bank, undated-a), China has become the world's second largest economy. Its growing wealth has lifted 680 million people out of poverty, accounting for 94 percent of the decline in poverty in developing countries (Tuck, 2013). Its life expectancy at birth increased from 44 years in 1961 to 73 years in 2011 (World Bank, undated-b). But rapid industrialization has had profound implications for the health care needs of the population. The confluence of urbanization, changes in lifestyle (including diet and physical activity), and population aging have led to what health researchers call the epidemiological transition from acute to chronic disease.

After having successfully expanded health insurance coverage, China now faces the challenge of building an effective and efficient delivery system to serve its large and aging population. The country finds itself at a crossroads—it can emulate the models of Western countries with their well-known limitations, or embark on an ambitious endeavor to create an innovative and sustainable model. In this report, we argue that China should choose the second option and design and implement a health care system based on population health management (PHM) principles and sophisticated health information technology (IT). Taking this path could yield a triple dividend for China: Health care will contribute to the growth of service sector employment, stimulate domestic demand by unlocking savings, and enable China to export its health system development capabilities to other countries, mirroring its success in building other critical infrastructure. Furthermore, improved access to affordable, high-quality care may diminish social unrest—a major concern of the Chinese government, and part of the impetus for launching one of several recent health care reform efforts (Tanner, 2005; Yip et al., 2012). These forces can help turn the Chinese Dream into a reality.

1.1. Research Approach

Our research is based on a review and synthesis of the peer-reviewed and gray literature, analysis of publicly available data sources, and expert interviews. We covered information on population trends, burden of disease, and demand for health care services in China, as well as data and publication on China's health care delivery infrastructure and workforce. We reviewed policy documents and position statements by Chinese officials, international organizations, and nongovernmental experts. Based on the findings of our review, we identified seminal publications to guide the development of our recommendation for China's future health care system.

1.2 Population Aging, Lifestyle Changes, and Growing Wealth Are Increasing the Burden of Chronic Disease and Disability in China

China's Population Is Aging Rapidly

China's population has been aging rapidly. Over the past 13 years, the proportion of the population over the age of 65 has reached the highest level in the history of the country, and it continues to climb. Based on United Nations population projections, elderly people will account for almost 20 percent of China's total population by 2025, and that figure is expected to increase to 30 percent by 2050 (Figure 1.1). The proportion of elderly people in China will then be higher than in any of the high-income nations, as demonstrated by data from the Organization for Economic Cooperation and Development (OECD). At the rate that the average age is currently increasing, China will be the first nation in history to achieve the designation of being an aged society before

Figure 1.1
Age Distribution of China's Population, 1990–2050

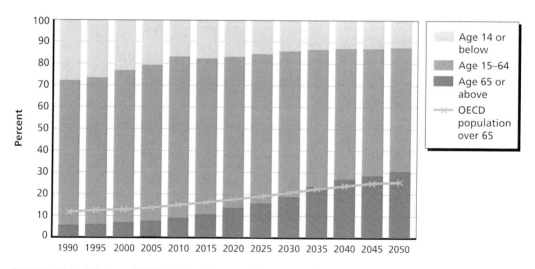

SOURCE: United Nations (2012); National Bureau of Statistics of China (2012).
NOTE: Populations of 2015–2050 are projections.
RAND RR600-1.1

it achieves the status of being a high-income country (defined by the World Bank as a country with a gross national income per capita of US$12,480 or more in 2011 dollars).

This aging population is one of the major challenges China will face in the coming decades. Thus, any approach to redesigning the health care system must begin with this demographic.

China Has Undergone Dramatic Social and Economic Changes

Over the past 30 years, economic reform has lifted millions of Chinese people out of poverty. Some 94 percent of the decline in poverty in developing countries during this time period can be credited to China (Tuck, 2013). This economic transformation and the social changes that have accompanied it have led to dramatic alterations in health-related behaviors and in people's risks for a variety of diseases, both acute and chronic.

Income growth, along with a surge in the food supply and in the variety of foods grown and imported, has significantly reduced the prevalence of malnutrition over the past 20 years. However, this rapidly evolving food environment has begun to have detrimental effects on health.

For instance, improvements in agricultural production and increased imports have resulted in major shifts in the typical pattern of nutrient intake. The World Bank reported in 2011 that, whereas the traditional Chinese diet contained only about 15 percent total fat and provided negligible amounts of sugar, the average fat content of the Chinese diet between 1982 and 2002 increased from 25 to 35 percent in urban areas and from 14 percent to 28 percent in rural areas (Centers for Disease Control and Prevention, 2013). Consumption of sugar-sweetened soft drinks in China has also increased (Wang, Marquez, and Langenbrunner, 2011). Both of these factors have contributed to rising rates of obesity across China.

Adding to the effects of dietary abundance, improved public transportation and longer work days have resulted in more than 16 percent of the population reporting a decrease in their activity levels (National Bureau of Statistics of China, 2007).

Finally, some 39 percent of the Chinese population smokes tobacco, almost twice the OECD average. The prevalence of smoking among Chinese men ages 15–69 is among the highest in the world (Wang, Marquez, and Langenbrunner, 2011).

These changes in dietary patterns, exercise behaviors, tobacco use, and other health-related behaviors have altered the prevalence of risk factors for noncommunicable, or chronic, diseases (NCDs). Over the past 20 years, rates of hypertension, elevated cholesterol, hyperglycemia, and overweight and obesity have been increasing significantly. Although cholesterol levels and body mass index (BMI, an indicator of weight status) remain lower in China than in OECD countries, the prevalence of hypertension by 2008 already exceeded the OECD average by almost 10 percentage points (Figure 1.2)

The changes in risk factors have resulted in substantial increases in NCDs. In 2008, NCDs accounted for 7,998,800, or 83 percent, of all deaths in China (World

Figure 1.2
Trends in Metabolic Risk Factors in China, 2008

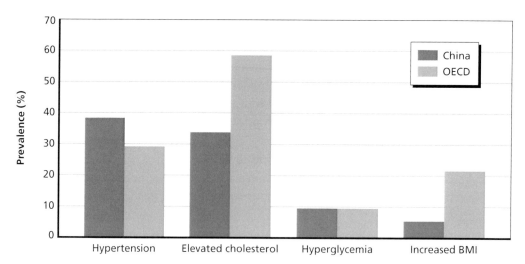

SOURCES: World Health Organization (2011); World Health Organization Global Health Observatory (2008).
RAND *RR600-1.2*

Figure 1.3
Prevalence of Noncommunicable Disease in China and OECD Countries

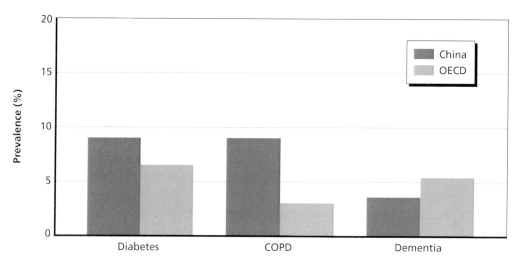

SOURCES: Fang, Wang, and Bai (2011); Organization for Economic Cooperation Development (2011, 2012a, 2012b); and Zhang et al. (2012).
RAND *RR600-1.3*

Figure 1.4
Mortality of Major Noncommunicable Diseases in China and OECD Countries

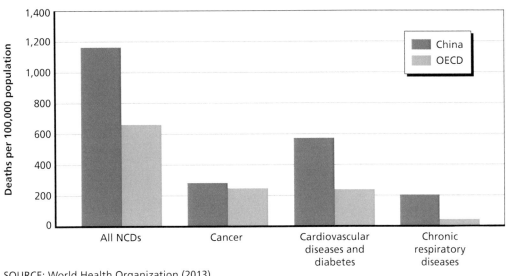

SOURCE: World Health Organization (2013).
RAND *RR600-1.4*

Health Organization, 2011). The World Health Organization projects that between 2010 and 2030, more than 100 million Chinese will die of a chronic disease, and that from 2005 to 2015, deaths from chronic diseases will increase by 19 percent; notably, deaths related to diabetes are expected to increase by 50 percent (World Health Organization, 2005). Compared to OECD countries, China has a higher proportion of people who suffer from diabetes and from chronic obstructive pulmonary disease (COPD) (see Figure 1.3). Mortality rates due to NCDs are higher in China than in OECD countries such as Japan, the United States, and the United Kingdom (Figure 1.4).

1.3. The Capacity of the Current Health Care Delivery System and Human Resource Pools Are Not Prepared to Meet the Increasing Demand for Public Health and Health Care Services

The emerging epidemic of NCDs combined with the rapid aging of the population imposes a significant burden not only on the health of the Chinese people (especially for low-income populations within China) but also on its health care system. While China can meet population needs for services such as maternal care, prenatal care, and childhood vaccinations, particularly in urban areas (Liu et al., 2008), its delivery system is not equipped to prevent and manage chronic diseases effectively (Wang, Marquez, and Langenbrunner, 2011).

China's Health Care System

Finance

Nearly the entire population has insurance through one of three plans recently created by the government:

Insurance plans	Year Launched	Description
Urban Employee Basic Medical Insurance (UEBMI)	1998	• For employed urban residents • Private and state-owned enterprises contribute • Beneficiaries responsible for about 1/3 of total inpatient costs
New Cooperative Medical Scheme (NCMS)	2003	• For rural residents • Central and local governments contribute • Beneficiaries responsible for more than 1/2 of total inpatient expenditures and about 2/3 of total outpatient expenditures
Urban Resident Basic Medical Insurance (URBMI)	2007	• For unemployed urban residents, including children and the elderly • Central and local governments contribute • Beneficiaries responsible for more than 1/2 of total inpatient expenditures and about 2/3 of total outpatient expenditures

- While insurance is nearly universal, cost-sharing remains high.
- Government subsidies comprise only about 10 percent of hospitals' total operating revenue. Payments for patient care make up the remainder of the revenue.
- Prices are regulated. The government has set prices for basic health care below cost, while setting high-tech diagnostic services above cost and allowing health care facilities a 15-percent profit margin on medicines.
- In public hospitals, physicians are employees, but they can receive bonuses for bringing in high levels of revenue for the hospitals.

Delivery

- Public-sector providers account for about 94 percent of all hospital admissions and about 81 percent of outpatient visits.
- In urban areas, care is delivered in community health centers (about 20 beds), secondary hospitals (100–499 beds), and tertiary hospitals (500+ beds). In rural areas, care is delivered in village clinics (a handful of beds), township health centers (about 20 beds), and county hospitals (100–499 beds).
- Due largely to patients' low trust in clinics and health centers, about 90 percent of health care services are delivered in hospitals.

SOURCES: Eggleston (2012); Meng and Tang (2010); "What can be learned from China's health system?" (2012); Yip et al. (2010); Yip et al. (2012); Yip and Hsiao (2008).

Several features of the current system prevent it from being well-equipped to respond to an aging population and rising rates of NCDs (see related text box for an overview of the finance and delivery systems in China). While most of the population has insurance through one of three plans that the government created in the past two decades, cost-sharing remains high, limiting citizens' access to care (Yip et al., 2012). Furthermore, in an effort to make care affordable while ensuring sufficient revenue for providers, the government set prices for basic health care below cost, while setting high-tech diagnostic services above cost and permitting a 15-percent profit margin on medicines (Yip and Hsiao, 2008). Consequently, China's health care payment system incentivizes the provision of high-tech care over preventive and disease management services. For a population increasingly burdened by NCDs, these services are crucial.

About 90 percent of health care is delivered in hospitals, with little care taking place in community health centers and village clinics that may be better equipped to provide preventive care and NCD management, as well as being less costly (What can be learned from China's health system? 2012). In addition, although the demand for health care services in China is comparable to that of OECD countries and the health care system has grown rapidly in the past several decades, the supply of health care professionals (e.g., physicians and nurses), as well as the number of hospital beds, remains inadequate (Yip and Hsiao, 2008). Compared with the OECD countries' 3.1 certified physicians and 8.6 registered nurses per 1,000 residents, China employs 1.6 physicians and 1.5 nurses per 1,000 people (Figure 1.5). Thus, the shortage of nurses in China

Figure 1.5
Number of Physicians and Nurses per Thousand Population in China and OECD Countries, 2005–2010

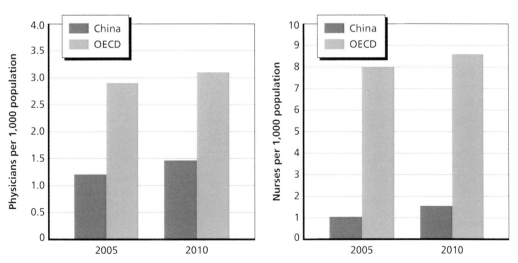

SOURCES: National Bureau of Statistics of China (2006; 2012) and Organization for Economic Cooperation Development (2012a).
RAND RR600-1.5

Figure 1.6
Number of Hospital Beds per Thousand Population in China and OECD Countries, 2005–2010

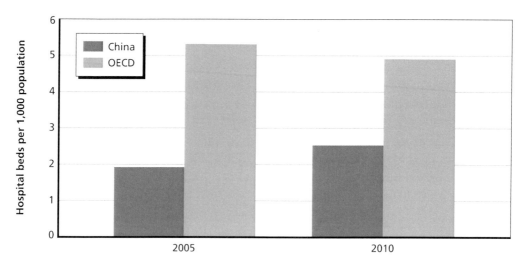

SOURCES: National Bureau of Statistics of China (2006; 2012) and Organization for Economic Cooperation Development (2012a).
RAND *RR600-1.6*

is even more severe than the shortage of physicians. The number of hospital beds per 1,000 residents is 2.6 in China, about half of that in OECD countries (Figure 1.6).

1.4. Building Capacity and Capabilities to Handle Expected Demand Remains a Challenge

To meet the current and projected demand for physicians in China, medical schools will need to increase capacity substantially. But recent efforts to increase enrollment by 30 percent have revealed a shortage of faculty, laboratory infrastructure, and other needed resources, suggesting that the capacity to expand enrollment further is limited. Given the current training capacity, and assuming medical student graduation and physician workforce exit rates remain unchanged (see Figure 1.7), it will take China about 21 years to reach the 2010 supply level of OECD countries (3.1 physicians per 1,000 residents). Put another way, training capacity would need to grow by 2.85 percent annually to reach the OECD level by 2020, which would be a challenging task given that the current capacity has already been exhausted. The government's current projections suggest that capacity is not likely to reach the needed level in the near future; projected rates are for 2.34 physicians and physician assistants per 1,000 residents by the year 2020, far below the 2010 rates of the OECD countries.

Figure 1.7
Number of Medical School Enrollees and Graduates per 1,000 Population in China, 2001–2010

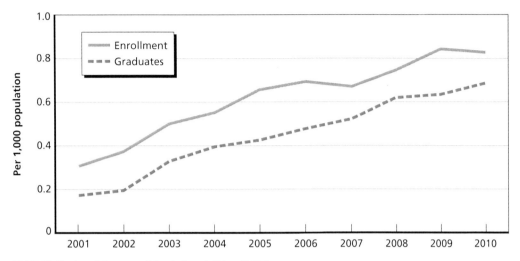

SOURCE: National Bureau of Statistics of China (2011).
RAND *RR600-1.7*

1.5. The Current System Has Limited Absorptive Capacity

A system's ability to expand to accommodate growing needs may be limited not by inadequate access to capital, but by the limited ability of institutions to make use of resources; that is, the ability to expand may be limited by a system's absorptive capacity. Research by the World Bank has confirmed this phenomenon (Burnside and Dollar, 2004; De Renzio, 2009; Hanson et al., 2003). Factors cited as potential limitations to the growth of health care services include a shortage of health care personnel, a lack of training facilities, and limits to the management and planning capabilities that are needed to oversee investments and to plan, build, and populate the facilities.

CHAPTER TWO

Designing and Implementing an Innovative Model for Organizing and Delivering Health Care Can Turn This Challenge into an Opportunity

2.1. Health Care as a Cornerstone of a Knowledge-Based Economy

China's current five-year plan calls for a transition from an economy focused on labor and natural resources to one that is knowledge-based; that is, an economy for which the creation and use of knowledge are central to economic development (Nolte et al., 2012). China's rapid development over the past three decades has transformed the country, lifting huge swaths of the population out of poverty. Now, the central government has seized on the opportunity to develop high-value modern industries with advanced technologies and large employment capacity. Recent data on the contribution of the manufacturing and service sectors to China's GDP (see Figure 2.1) show that China has already begun to move in this direction; in fact, in the first quarter of

Figure 2.1
Contribution of Manufacturing and Service Sectors to GDP in China, 2006–2013

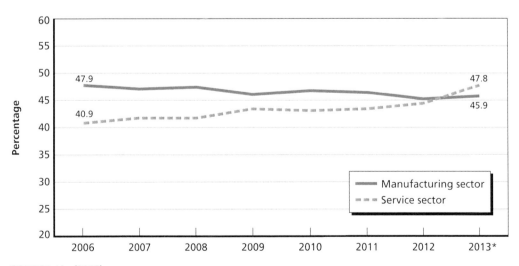

SOURCE: Liu (2013)
NOTE: *2013 first quarter data only.
RAND RR600-2.1

2013, the service sector exceeded the manufacturing sector in contributions to GDP for the first time.

As with other countries that have reached this point of development, China's health care industry promises to be a cornerstone of its desired transition to a knowledge-based economy. In developed countries, health care is one of the largest segments of the service sector, accounting for between 7 percent and 16 percent of the economy—and in OECD countries, average spending on health care as a percentage of GDP is above 9 percent. Health care expenditures in China have increased over the past three decades to 5 percent of GDP; thus the potential for growth remains great.

In developed countries, the health care sector employs a sizable proportion of the population. In the United States, for example, about 10 percent of the employed population works in this sector (Center for Sustainable Health Spending, 2013). Importantly, the health care sector has been resilient in the face of the recent severe recession, growing by almost 11 percent from late 2007 to early 2013 as the rest of employment shrank by more than 3 percent (Center for Sustainable Health Spending, 2013). Since China's current five-year plan calls for the creation of 45 million new jobs, rapid development of the health care sector is an effective way to achieve—and sustain—this employment goal and a powerful engine to promote domestic consumption, further transforming the current investment-heavy economy.

2.2. Unlocking Savings to Increase Domestic Demand

China has long recognized the need to transition from an export-driven economy to one with greater domestic consumption. In fact, this transition is one of the key goals identified in the five-year plan. China's famously high growth rates of the past few decades have not been matched by growth in consumption. At more than 30 percent, China's average household savings rate is one of the highest in the world, and has actually increased since the mid-1990s, when it was less than 20 percent (Barnett, Myrvoda, and Nabar, 2012). The Chinese government is rightfully concerned about the high rate of savings, because it depresses the domestic consumption necessary to reduce dependence on exports.

The growth in the savings rate in China appears attributable, in part, to the private burden of health expenditures; as families anticipate having to pay out of pocket for a high share of their medical care, they save a substantial portion of their income as a precautionary measure (Chamon and Prasad, 2008; Cristadoro and Marconi, 2012). With greater access to health insurance and decreased copayments, the Chinese people might be freed to save a smaller proportion of their incomes, increasing consumption rates and supporting the transition from an export-driven economy. In fact, research suggests that for every yuan increase in Chinese government health care spending in urban areas, household savings decrease by two yuan (Brooks and Barnett, 2010).

Thus, improving access to health care presents a remarkable opportunity for the government to stimulate economic growth through increased domestic demand.

2.3. Successful Innovative Models Stimulates Export of Services and Capabilities to Develop and Maintain Critical Infrastructure

As developing countries grow wealthier and undergo the transition to a burden of care needs dominated by NCDs, they will seek a health care system that meets these new needs. However, few health care systems in the developed world are organized and financed to meet the population's needs cost-effectively. The absence of appropriate models creates a significant opportunity for a country like China. If China is able to transition to a health care system that is tailored to the demands of the 21st century and reflective of technological progress, it can develop the capability to offer health system development to other countries (or private enterprise within other countries), mirroring its success in building other critical infrastructure, such as for transportation and energy, abroad.

Indeed, over the past 15 years or so, the global market for the development of infrastructure such as service-sector industries has grown (Yescombe, 2011). Public-private partnerships, in which a government contracts with a domestic or foreign company for infrastructure development, are increasingly popular in both developing and developed countries (Yescombe, 2011). If China successfully implements an innovative health care system, it will be well positioned to create a new export industry of health care infrastructure and services, thereby catalyzing a wave of economic growth.

CHAPTER THREE

The "Western-Style" Health Care Model Offers Cautionary Lessons for China

Many experts have noted the mismatch between the health care needs of 21st-century societies and the way health care is organized, financed, and delivered in mature economies, which we refer to in this report as the "Western-style" model of health care. This model evolved in an era dominated by conditions that required acute care for conditions such as infections, injuries, and childbirth. The health care delivery systems, multilevel infrastructure for financing care, and even the predominant paradigm for innovation were shaped by that historical context. Thus, if one imagines the demand for health care as a pyramid, with the top representing high-tech care for acute health problems (such as cardiac surgery and bone marrow transplantation), and the bottom representing maintenance of the health, wellness, and productivity of the population, countries employing a Western-style model have devoted a disproportionately large share of resources and leadership attention to the top and are getting poor value for the money.

Though many countries exhibit the undesirable characteristics of the Western-style model, the United States offers a particularly stark example, as it spends more than $8,000 per person annually—about 17.5 percent of its GDP or almost twice as much as the OECD average (Kaiser Family Foundation, 2013). The United States epitomizes the Western-style health care model, with a system that lacks continuity and coordination but overuses expensive diagnostic and therapeutic options. As a result, the United States performs poorly on many measures of health care quality while having high spending levels.

While China has incorporated effective components of the Western model, such as social insurance, other components present barriers to meeting the needs of 21st-century societies: limited IT investment, a lack of adherence to evidence-based practices in clinical care, limited performance monitoring and improvement efforts, encounter-based care, poor coordination among providers, misaligned incentives, and lack of consumer involvement. These aspects of the Western model—and the experiences of countries that are attempting to reform them—offer valuable lessons to countries, like China, that are dedicated to developing high-performing health care systems.

3.1. Limited Investment in Information Technology Relative to Other Industries

During the IT "revolution" of the late 20th century, many industries invested substantially in IT, achieving efficiency gains (Kaiser Family Foundation, 2013). By contrast, health care providers have been slow to adopt IT, and governments have struggled to stimulate uptake. Even after the RAND Corporation published widely cited research in 2005 suggesting that health IT could produce $81 billion in annual savings for the United States (Hillestad et al., 2005), hospitals and ambulatory centers have been slow to adopt, with just 40 percent of physician practices and 27 percent of hospitals meeting the standards for "basic" electronic health records (Kellermann and Jones, 2013). A few countries, such as the Netherlands, the United Kingdom, and Australia, have been successful in achieving nearly universal use of electronic health records (EHRs) in ambulatory practices. However, even in these countries, adoption of EHRs in hospitals remains limited (Jha et al., 2008).

Discouragingly, hospitals and physician practices that have invested in health IT hoping to improve efficiency and outcomes have found their ability to utilize these technologies seriously impeded by interoperability issues. In the United States, hospitals and ambulatory practices have many health IT systems and vendors to choose from. And even when different providers purchase the same system from the same vendor, the systems are customized to each provider's needs to the point where they are no longer interoperable and unable to talk to each other. Since a key reason for installing such systems in the first place is to improve coordination of care across different providers, this lack of interoperability is a major limitation.

The United Kingdom: Maximizing General Practitioners' Use of EHRs
In the last decade, the government of the United Kingdom has undertaken two sizable initiatives aimed at increasing the effective use of health IT. First, the government has directly supported purchase and maintenance of EHRs (Jha et al., 2008). Second, the government included measures of the use of EHR features, such as clinical decision support, in its pay-for-performance scheme for general practitioners (Jha, et al., 2008) (for more on this, see Chapter Four). These efforts have been recognized as contributing to EHR adoption and use (Berthold et al., 2011; Jha et al., 2008). In fact, the United Kingdom now has one of the highest rates of EHR use worldwide among general practitioners, with more than 90 percent of general practitioners using EHRs.

3.2. Lack of Adherence to Guidelines and Best Practices

Clinical practice guidelines synthesize the best available evidence about the appropriate treatment for patients with a specific condition to improve quality of care and standardize practice. Clinicians, as well as hospital managers, payers, and health system planners, can use clinical practice guidelines to inform their decisionmaking about care for individual patients or groups of patients. The past few decades have seen a proliferation of such guidelines: As of 2011, the Guidelines International Network contained more than 3,700 clinical practices guidelines from 39 countries (Institute of Medicine, 2011). Despite the growing number of guidelines, research in many countries (including Canada, Australia, and the United States) suggests that physicians typically do not follow such guidelines (Cabana et al., 1999). Key barriers include lack of awareness of guidelines, disagreement with recommendations, and the perception that guidelines are inconvenient or difficult to use (Cabana et al., 1999).

3.3. Limited Performance Monitoring and Improvement

Traditionally, societies have relied on the medical profession to ensure quality of care through self-regulation and have not interfered with clinical autonomy, but research over the past two decades has cast doubt over the viability of this arrangement (Mattke, 2004). For example, a 1999 report by the National Academy of Sciences' Institute of Medicine (an independent research organization) estimated that between 44,000 and 98,000 people die in the United States each year due to preventable medical errors (Institute of Medicine, 1999).

In response, governments and health care system managers are increasingly undertaking efforts to measure quality, as well as other aspects of care, such as efficiency and patient experience. For example, the OECD has developed performance indicators through the Health Care Quality Indicator Project with the intention of comparing quality across OECD countries (Arah et al., 2006). Governments and other payers have also implemented programs that aim to hold providers accountable for performance. In Germany, the Federal Office for Quality Assurance (BQS) monitors hospital performance on 194 measures, summarizing its findings in reports to individual hospitals. Hospitals that are found to be underperforming must explain their performance to BQS and, in some cases, take actions to improve it (Busse, Nimptsch, and Mansky, 2009). In the United Kingdom, about 20 percent of primary care providers' income is related to their performance on quality indicators (Doran et al., 2006).

3.4 Physician-Centric, Encounter-Based, and Poorly Coordinated Care

In the past, care delivery occurred mostly during actual encounters of patients with physicians and other care providers. As a result, a payment system evolved that links remuneration or revenue to such encounters. This system both reflects and reinforces the focus on encounter-based care. However, as societies undergo a demographic transition toward a higher burden of chronic disease, the limitations of this model become apparent.

As payment is tied to the encounters, and not to any other activities, the workflow is established in a way that requires a physician to make all relevant decisions during an office visit. This setup is efficient if all relevant decisions *can* be made during an encounter, as is the case for many acute problems, but fails to provide ongoing care for patients with chronic disease. Experts attest that having more patient-care activities take place outside of office visits is likely to improve quality, save time, and reduce costs. Patients with chronic disease require ongoing monitoring between encounters (as well as support and coordination services) as they transition from one care setting to the next, such as from a hospital back to the home.

In the United States and elsewhere, alternative payment and delivery arrangements—such as paying providers on a capitated basis (i.e., a set fee per patient) with a bonus for good health outcomes—have been introduced with the intent of supporting the provision of care outside of face-to-face encounters, as well as the coordination of care. However, several factors, such as the large body of stakeholders that benefit from the status quo, make reforms like these challenging to implement (Chen et al., 2011). These factors are further explored in Chapter Four.

Systems that revolve around physician-patient encounters tend to be physician-centric at the expense of team-based care and task-shifting. Experts emphasize that the complex needs of chronically ill patients require the collaboration of multidisciplinary health care teams—including, for example, primary care physicians, nurses, nutritionists, rehabilitation specialists, and social workers, which are infrequently used. A few particularly innovative health care delivery organizations, such as Kaiser Permanente, based in California (in the United States), have created training programs and workflows that maximize the use of multidisciplinary teams (Bodenheimer, Chen, and Bennett, 2009). However, the majority of delivery organizations do not employ this approach, and in the United States, projections suggest that the health care workforce of the future will not be capable of forming such teams in sufficient numbers (Bodenheimer, Chen, and Bennett, 2009).

Another consequence of tying payment to encounters and procedures is the emergence of so-called silos. Health care funds are often budgeted by sector, such as inpatient care, ambulatory care, and prescription drugs. This practice can create disincentives against aligning care delivery with patient needs. For example, a global survey on home health care technology revealed that home monitoring after hospital discharge continues to be underused because hospitals tend to get paid for additional admissions but not for avoidance of readmissions. Thus, the hospital would have to bear the cost of monitoring patients after discharge while forgoing the revenue of a readmission. Singapore's health care system offers another example: This system has optimized access to acute care through public clinics and access to hospital care in subsidized facilities but provides only limited insurance coverage and coordination for chronic care needs, resulting in fragmented and poor quality care (Lee, 2008).

Some developing countries are following the ill-advised lead of the United States and other countries with Western-style health care. This year, Myanmar's Ministry of Health released plans to build four new 500-bed hospitals in the capital, Nay Pyi Taw (Myanmar Phar-med Expo 2013, 2013). Remarkably, in response to criticism about this development, which was widely perceived as unnecessary, the Ministry of Health acknowledged the lack of demand for new hospitals and decided to reallocate the funds to work on an existing hospital and the development of a medical school. Anecdotally, several Middle Eastern states that have built large hospitals find it difficult to attract specialty physicians and sufficient patient volumes for those facilities.

Delivery System Reform: Germany's Efforts to Improve Coordination

Over the past two decades, Germany's government has embarked on several efforts to improve care coordination, especially for patients with chronic diseases (Nolte et al., 2012). For example, hospitals have been allowed to provide outpatient care since 1993; prior to this reform, only office-based physicians were paid to provide ambulatory services (U.S. Congress, 1995). As a result, hospitals started offering preoperative management and care transition services after discharge. In 2003, the German government introduced disease management programs that support evidence-based practice and increased coordination for patients with chronic diseases (Busse, 2004). Providers that join these programs are eligible for additional payments, if they meet standards for care coordination and use of team-based care (Miksch et al., 2010; Szecsenyi, Rosemann, and Joos, 2008). Disease management programs have become the norm for the care of several chronic diseases in Germany (Blumel & Busse, 2009), with positive results. For example, patient participation in diabetes management programs has been associated with reduced mortality (Miksch et al., 2010).

3.5. Misaligned Incentives

Encounter-based payment creates incentives for providers to conduct additional services, which can lead to overuse. Not only can overuse waste resources (IMS Institute
for Healthcare Informatics, 2013), but it also threatens patient safety.

The wasted resources that result from overuse are especially a cause for concern
when they involve high-cost and high-margin services, such as diagnostic imaging and
discretionary surgery. And even when scientific evidence discourages use of services
and/or expensive drugs, practice patterns often change slowly (Timbie et al., 2012).

Overuse also threatens patient safety—for example, through exposure to radiation during discretionary imaging or through potential complications from invasive
procedures. The Institute of Medicine defines overuse as "the provision of care for
which the potential risks outweigh the potential benefits" (Institute of Medicine Committee on Quality of Health Care in America, 2001). Several decades of research have
demonstrated that overuse is a substantial problem in health care, and two areas of
research in particular have quantified its magnitude.

Researchers at Dartmouth University discovered the phenomenon of geographic
variation in the rates of use of a broad range of common medical procedures, including
cesarean sections, magnetic resonance imaging, and heart surgery (Darmouth Institute for Health Policy and Clinical Practice, 2012). They showed that variation is much
higher than could be explained by variation in patient need, and also that use patterns
are inconsistent (i.e., a region could have high rates for one procedure but low rates for
another).

Accountable Care Organizations in the United States: Aligning Incentives for Lower-Cost, Higher-Quality Care

The 2010 health care reform legislation in the United States prioritized
payment reform to create incentives for higher quality care and lower costs.
One major component of this effort was the creation of accountable care
organizations (ACOs)—provider-led organizations with a strong primary
care component, in which part of the payment is linked to care quality and
efficiency. While an ACO is paid on a fee-for-service schedule, it is held
accountable for the overall cost of care: Expected medical costs of providing
care for its assigned population are estimated with statistical models. If the
ACO manages to hold cost below the projection, it receives a share of the
estimated savings (Berwick, 2011). In addition, ACOs need to meet targets
for quality standards, such as adequate blood glucose control in its diabetic
patients and agreed-upon targets for member satisfaction. Since the reform
was passed, more than 300 organizations have become ACOs, covering about
10 percent of the population (Fisher, 2013).

The second area of research on variation in medical decisionmaking and use of procedures is the appropriateness research that originated at RAND (Brook, 1995). This research uses evidence and expert opinion to define explicit criteria to judge the appropriateness of a variety of medical procedures given a particular patient's symptoms, comorbidities, and diagnostic findings. Using the results of such appropriateness investigations, researchers typically find that about a third of high-cost, high-risk procedures, such as carotid surgery or cardiac catheterization, are performed in patients without an appropriate indication.

3.6 Lack of Consumer Involvement in Care

Health care providers and systems have been criticized for insufficiently engaging patients in decisions about their health care (Coulter, 1999). Several factors contribute to this tendency, including paternalism and payment systems that favor procedures over time spent with patient education. As a result, patients lack sufficient understanding of their conditions and the importance of treatment plan adherence and self-management (National eHealth Collaborative, 2010). A recent review summarized the evidence for the relationship between patient engagement and activation and outcomes, and stated that activated patients tend to have better health outcomes, better experience of care, and lower cost (Hibbard and Greene, 2013).

CHAPTER FOUR

Fast-Growing Economies Like China's Have a Unique Opportunity to Implement Innovative Health Care Systems

In countries with Western-style health care systems, concern is growing about the health outcomes and financial sustainability of these systems, leading to calls for fundamental reform. However, reform efforts are often thwarted by what political scientists call *path dependence*; i.e., situations in which policymakers' options are constrained by history and existing institutional structures. Established health care systems tend to have many entrenched stakeholders who are familiar with and benefit from the status quo and who resist change unless fully compensated. As a consequence, policymakers are often unable to reform policies—even if they realize the current system does not achieve optimal outcomes—or are able to effect change only if they offer substantial compensation to existing stakeholders. By contrast, rapidly growing economies such as China's have an advantage when it comes to reforming their health care systems: To a larger degree than long-established health systems with significant path dependence, China has the opportunity to design its health care systems de novo, as greater wealth allows for increasing access to care. This situation is akin to the conditions that promoted Germany's *Wirtschaftswunder* (economic miracle) in the 1950s. The destruction wrought by World War II and the dismantling of key industries by the allied forces had nearly eliminated Germany's industrial base. But a rapid influx of capital allowed the country to invest in state-of-the-art manufacturing facilities and quickly outpace countries burdened with legacy infrastructure.

The difficulties that policymakers face when trying to reform established health care systems can be illustrated by many examples. Various attempts to implement health care reform in the United States are particularly familiar. While the world's largest economy has long spent more than any other country on health care as a share of its wealth, it has been unable to provide universal health care coverage: About 15 percent of the population has no health care coverage (Centers for Disease Control and Prevention, 2012). Several attempts to achieve universal coverage have failed over the past 20 years. For example, President Bill Clinton's Health Security Act, a 1993 proposal to expand insurance coverage and impose stronger regulations on the health care industry to improve cost controls, was heavily attacked by interest groups, particularly the powerful insurance industry. In the end, the proposal did not get enough support from

Clinton's own Democratic Party to be voted on, and the bill was abandoned (Skocpol, 1997).

In 2010, President Barack Obama was able to pass a major health reform bill with the Patient Protection and Affordable Care Act, which will substantially expand coverage. However, interest groups had extensive involvement in shaping the content of this legislation (Quadagno, 2011). The private insurance industry, employers, trade unions, pharmaceutical and medical device companies, health care provider groups, and other organizations invested heavily in lobbying members of Congress to include or exclude specific provisions (Quadagno, 2011; Steinbrook, 2009). In fact, more than eight lobbyists per member of Congress were hired to influence the health care reform effort in 2009 (Eaton and Pell, 2011). In 2009 and 2010, more than $1 billion was spent lobbying on behalf of health care reform in the United States (Liberto, 2011). As a result, the eventual bill will expand health care coverage but will not, for the most part, introduce fundamental changes to the organization and delivery of health care, simply extending a costly system to more citizens.

Private health insurance companies in the United States face similar obstacles in attempting to encourage providers to make cost-saving changes in the way they deliver health care services. For example, private insurers are encouraging primary care providers to become so-called patient-centered medical homes, which would provide ongoing support and care coordination services for their patients, particularly those with chronic diseases. The rationale for patient-centered medical homes is that better support for chronically ill patients will prevent costly exacerbations, thus improving health outcomes and reducing costs. A recent systematic review, for example, found that, overall, patient-centered medical homes improve quality of care, reduce errors, and improve patient experiences (Rosenthal, 2008). A subsequent study reported a reduction in emergency room visits and hospital admissions, as well as overall cost savings, among patient-centered medical home patients (Fields, Leshen, and Patel, 2010). But to get providers to establish such delivery models, insurance companies realized they had to offer financial incentives, so that the financial gains from improved care delivery may largely accrue to providers.

Other countries with mature health care systems have faced similar difficulties in implementing health care reform. In 2000, South Korea's government passed legislation that would eliminate physicians' authority to sell medications directly to patients (Ahmad, 2000). Prior to this policy change, both physicians and pharmacists were authorized to prescribe *and* sell medications (Watts, 2001). Since physicians and pharmacists received income from medications they sold, they had a financial incentive to prescribe unneeded medications (Watts, 2001). This overprescribing resulted in antibiotic resistance and abuse of medications (Kim and Ruger, 2008; Watts, 2001). To align incentives with the needs of patients, as opposed to the financial interests of physicians and pharmacists, the South Korean government decided to limit the authority of doctors and pharmacists such that doctors are only able to prescribe medications and pharmacists are only able to sell and dispense (Watts, 2001). Physicians, having had prescribing authority for years, went on strike (Ahmad, 2000), closing 80 percent of medical clinics in the country ("Doctors' protest hobbles health care," February 18, 2000). After six days of strikes during which a number of deaths were attributed to the absence of working physicians, the government agreed to increase physician fees for medical consultations by 72 percent and to increase fees for prescribing medications by 500 percent (Kim and Ruger, 2008). These higher fees were covered by a 21-percent increase in worker health insurance contributions (Watts, 2001). As is often seen in countries with established health care systems, needed reform came at a high price; in South Korea, the government achieved its goal of separating medication prescribing from selling but failed to realize the expected spending decrease (Kim and Ruger, 2008).

In 2004, the National Health Service in the United Kingdom undertook an ambitious initiative to shift payment for primary care toward rewarding better performance (NHS Employers, 2013; Scottish Government, 2011). Primary care physicians (called general practitioners, or GPs) work under contract with the National Health Service and are mostly paid on a capitated basis, with some additional payments for selected services and capital and IT (Smith and York, 2004). When the National Health Service negotiated a new GP contract in 2004, one key element was the introduction of payments associated with the performance of primary care practices on a complex set of 146 quality measures (Lester et al., 2006) that focus on chronic disease management and practice organization (Charlton, 2005). But GPs negotiated protection for their previous compensation and bonus payments for performance on the quality measures (Charlton, 2005). In the three subsequent years, GPs' average income increased by about 50 percent to £110,000 (US$224,400) (Cockcroft, 2007). Furthermore, any improvement in the quality measures that followed implementation of the new system was judged to be modest at best (Gillam, 2011).

Compared with countries that have long-established health care systems, China's post-economic reform system remains relatively unburdened by existing arrangements, infrastructure, and entrenched stakeholders. China has to choose between emulating the Western-style model with the flaws we have discussed and establishing an innovative model to meet the future needs of its aging population (what we call the PHM model). Because China is committed to substantially increasing spending on health care, this change can be communicated to stakeholders as an opportunity rather than a threat to their livelihood.

CHAPTER FIVE

Adopting Population Health Management Can Propel China to World-Class Health Care

In the wake of the miraculous economic growth that China experienced during the past several decades, the forces of rapid modernization and development combined with the accelerating aging of the population have dramatically increased its burden of chronic disease. Our analysis points to a substantial gap between China's current health care infrastructure and workforce and the demand for care, and suggests that the gaps will continue to widen. The speed at which the burden of chronic disease is growing, combined with China's vast population, imply that scaling up the existing health care system and bolstering its workforce through training or immigration will not be sufficient to meet demand.

At the same time, given its rapid economic and societal development, China occupies a unique position, even among large modernizing countries, in having the opportunity to build a world-class health care system from the ground up, relatively free of the entrenched stakeholders that hold back the health care systems of most developed and many developing countries.

We recommend that China build a new model that has not existed in its entirety but that incorporates effective pieces of other models. This new model would be built on PHM principles and operated with industrial principles of process optimization and use of advanced IT. Doing so would avoid other countries' mistakes and enable China to achieve Donald Berwick's concept of the *Three-Part Aim*: better care quality and patient experience, better population health, and lower costs (Berwick, Nolan, and Whittington, 2008).

5.1. A Blueprint for China's Future Health Care System

We would argue that China's future health care system should follow two design principles: one centered on human capital and the other focused on population health. First, to cope with the relative shortage of health care professionals, China needs to leverage highly skilled workers through sophisticated health IT and through shifting tasks to less-trained workers. In other words, routine and administrative tasks should be automated and delegated to the degree possible to allow scarce health care professionals, like physicians and nurses, to focus on complex tasks.

Second, China should adopt a PHM model, which unites the public health perspective of improving health at the population level and the medical care perspective of individual care delivery (Stoto, 2013). The defining characteristics of the PHM model are a focus on the health outcomes of the entire population; coordination of health and medical services through the continuum of care needs, from prevention and health promotion, to curative care, disease management and palliative care; and proactive management of care needs. A PHM model will be well equipped to address the future needs of an aging population that is experiencing an increased prevalence of health risk factors and the higher burden of disease and disability that results.

Elements of the PHM model can be found in reform efforts that many countries are currently undertaking, such as the *Selektivverträge* (selective contracting) between sickness funds and primary care practices in Germany, the Clinical Commissioning Groups in the United Kingdom, and the ACOs in the United States. Early results show that successful ACOs improved quality of care, decreased inpatient admissions, and reduced health care costs (Centers for Medicare and Medicaid Services, 2013). Importantly, Chinese leaders are recognizing the importance of care continuity: During the opening ceremony of the 18th Communist Party of China (CPC) National Congress, Hu Jintao, the former General Secretary of the Party, emphasized that China's health care delivery system should prioritize disease prevention, not just disease treatment (Hu, 2012), a principle congruent with that of PHM.

Our proposed blueprint for China's future health care systems has six interrelated components (Figure 5.1):

- sophisticated IT
- data-driven optimization of care processes
- performance monitoring at all levels of accountability
- effective deployment of health professionals
- aligned incentives
- consumer engagement.

Sophisticated Information Technology

A sophisticated IT infrastructure with robust capacity for expansion and adaptive innovation serves as the central cog for the envisioned PHM model because it will provide data and decision support that will be critically needed for all the other components. The infrastructure needs to have the following features:

- **structured content** that allows storage of critical data points as coded variables rather than as unstructured text

Figure 5.1
Blueprint for China's Future Health Care System

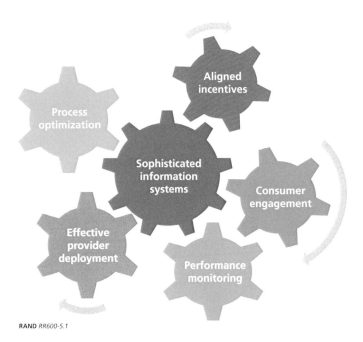

RAND *RR600-5.1*

- **a high degree of usability** to facilitate data entry and information retrieval, as well as clinical decision support, such as alerts for drug-drug interactions, diagnostic algorithms, and clinical order sets (Office of the National Coordinator for Health Information Technology, 2013)
- **interoperability** to allow data exchange between entities and different information systems
- **secure standards** for data access and transmission
- **role-based data access** to provide a window into the data that is customized for each user type. For example, individual clinicians would see a patient's trajectory; hospital managers would receive aggregate information on daily activities of all patients; and health systems planners would see aggregate information for their jurisdiction.
- **sufficient expandable capacity** to meet surges in user demand and avoid system crashes.

Complementing the sophisticated IT infrastructure will be a newly created professional called the health navigator. Given the shortage of providers, especially nurses, as well as the complexity involved in coordinating care across a broad range of providers and settings, health navigators will play a central role in our envisioned model. They will be paraprofessionals who are familiar with the entire health and health care systems, the care system's organization, and its operation, and who will be trained in basic clinical skills. Their role is not to provide care but to direct individuals assigned to them toward the most effective, efficient, and convenient sources of care, given their needs.

The navigator may identify and coordinate various resources, such as community-based health promotion and prevention activities, primary care, specialty care, inpatient care, emergency care, rehabilitative care, long-term care, and palliative care. As care needs will be determined by the decisions of clinicians and evidence-based algorithms coded into the IT system, navigators will require only basic clinical training. For example, a navigator who receives an alert that a diabetic patient does not adhere to her medications may refer her to pharmacist counseling, which does not require a deep understanding of disease biology and pharmacology. Similar roles exist in other systems: In the United States, discharge planners support patients in the transition from hospital to home and coordinate support services, such as home visits or delivery of meals. Together, sophisticated IT and health navigators could serve as an effective mechanism for meeting rapidly growing population needs in the absence of a sufficient supply of providers.

Building health IT infrastructure is an increasingly high priority in China. A recent country-wide reform plan identified medical informatics as one of the critical components of reform (Zhao et al., 2010). Several cities have initiated major efforts

Using the PHM Information Technology for Management Decisions—An Example

In February, Mrs. Wu, the operations manager at a large toy factory, was getting concerned about recent production delays because the factory had just received a large order from a new customer. Her line manager explained that an unusual number of workers had been out sick in the past few weeks, and overall performance was lagging. In response, Mrs. Wu requested a report on diagnoses for hospital admissions and clinic visits for her workforce from the local information exchange that houses all PHM data. The report, which listed only aggregated information to protect the workers' privacy, showed above-average rates for influenza and other respiratory illness in the previous weeks. Mrs. Wu asked the local health bureau for help; in response, the bureau sent an infectious disease nurse to the factory to discuss the report with her and her line managers. In the meeting, Mrs. Wu learned that the line managers had encouraged workers to take as few sick days as possible and work overtime, even if they did not feel well, because of the delays. The nurse explained that this advice was actually counterproductive, because sick workers would come to work and spread germs to their colleagues. She gave the line managers educational brochures and break-room posters to educate workers about hand washing, infection control, and staying home if feverish. Within four weeks, production was again running as scheduled.

to develop regional health care information sharing platforms that allow information sharing across hospitals within and between regions (Zhao et al., 2010). The sophisticated health IT infrastructure we have described would build off of this foundation.

Data-Driven Optimization of Care Processes

The IT infrastructure will allow the optimization of care delivery based on clinical evidence and best practices. In areas for which clear clinical evidence or sufficient consensus is available to guide decisions, clinical leaders can code those recommendations directly into the system in the form of decision algorithms and order sets. Where standards of care are still ambiguous, health services researchers can analyze differences in clinical decisions and correlate variations in practice with outcomes to develop a future evidence base. Similarly, managers can apply operations research tools and methods to optimize resource utilization decisions and provide guidance on efficient care delivery.

Performance Monitoring at All Levels of Accountability

As pointed out in Chapter Three, Western-style health care systems achieve low value for money, as outcomes are poor in spite of high levels of spending. We expect that robust IT can help health system planners and managers yield substantial gain in performance through:

- **benchmarking** clinical results and resource use against peer groups, such as other jurisdictions or institutions
- **investigating root causes** for areas of underperformance and devising remedial plans
- **identifying** top and bottom performers to derive and promulgate best practices.

This goal will be accomplished by constructing a comprehensive set of key performance indicators for technical quality of care, health outcomes, patient experience, and resource use at the lowest level of accountability (such as an individual physician or a care team) and then aggregating the indicators up to the respective level of decision-making. For example, the medical director of a clinic would receive reports on individual providers and for the entire clinic; the Health Bureau would receive reports on all clinics and at the level of its jurisdiction. Chinese leaders have indicated readiness to move in this direction; for example, former General Secretary Hu Jintao noted during the opening ceremony of the 18th CPC National Congress that monitoring provider performance should be a high priority for health care reform (Hu, 2012).

Having a rich data infrastructure will be the precondition for measuring the complex construct of clinical quality in a valid and credible way. For example, since a provider's outcomes depend not only on his or her decisions but also on the underlying risk of his or her patients, indicators must be adequately adjusted for patient mix to allow for fair comparisons, which requires detailed clinical data at the patient level. Similarly, providers and institutions should be held accountable only for outcomes that are under their control.

Ultimately, the performance monitoring system can be used for reporting performance to the public to encourage consumer choice and competition among providers, as well as pay-for-performance strategies for providers.

Effective Deployment of Health Professionals

Our analysis suggests that China has a shortage of medical professionals and insufficient training capacity to achieve staffing levels comparable to Western countries with a similar disease burden. However, it is not clear that China should emulate the Western-style staffing models and their traditionally heavy reliance on physicians. Rather, we expect that a combination of task shifting, increasing nurse training, and leveraging of health care staff in nonmedical settings can improve the capacity at current physician staffing levels.

Effective deployment of health professionals includes better task-shifting and "practicing at the top of one's license" (i.e., focusing on tasks that cannot be performed by professionals with a lower level of training or certification) and shifting tasks that can be performed by professionals or paraprofessionals with less training. For example, primary care physicians would concentrate on patients with complex chronic conditions, whereas advance practice nurses would see patients with routine complaints, such as sinusitis and minor injuries. Pharmacists would counsel on medication use and adherence, and health coaches would advise on health-related behaviors. Administrative and clerical tasks would be delegated to administrative assistants. Robust clinical decision support based on the IT we have discussed would expand the range of services that can safely and effectively be delegated and ensure that patient data are properly documented and shared.

At the same time, the information infrastructure allows involvement of a much broader range of health professionals in the care process because they can be made aware of patient needs and document their decisions and services to ensure proper coordination. For example, traditional Chinese medical practices can be integrated with Western care. Likewise, work and school-based professionals and local public health staff can be tasked to deliver preventive services.

Alignment of Incentives with Policy Goals

Experience with health care reform has demonstrated the importance of aligning incentives to obtain better care, better health outcomes, and lower costs. As Western countries are struggling to undo an incentive structure that has rewarded volume instead of value, China is in a unique position to introduce a sophisticated payment system, supported by IT, that steers providers and patients toward effective and prudent choices. Three main lessons emerge from our analysis:

- **Avoid payment silos.** A payment system that is organized by care setting creates disincentives to coordination and integration. For example, if hospitals are paid per admission, they have no financial rationale for investing in postdischarge care and care transition management. Instead, funds ought to follow the patient across settings.
- **Reward value, not volume.** The fee-for-service payment system is now viewed as a key obstacle to improving care, as it rewards providers for additional services, irrespective of clinical benefit. By contrast, a value-based payment system would reward a primary care physician (for example, for controlling the blood pressure and glucose level of diabetics).
- **Encourage prudent decisions.** While choice is important, patients need to have a certain degree of responsibility for their decisions and actions, both with respect to provider choice and lifestyle decisions.

On the supply side, a PHM system is, by definition, population-centric, and its payment system should cross care settings. Similarly, the same rules that are programmed into the health-information infrastructure to guide clinical decisions should be used to incentivize providers. A physician may choose to deviate from an evidence-based course of action to preserve clinical freedom, but the payment for this service will decrease.

On the demand side, China continues to have substantial cost-sharing requirements, and patients are not as isolated from their decisions as in other countries. But there is an opportunity to stratify cost-sharing requirements to steer patients toward choices that are consistent with policy goals and system performance. For example, services that can reduce overall cost, such as immunizations and medicines to control diabetes and blood pressure, could be offered to patients at no cost. Conversely, seeking care at high-intensity settings for minor problems could be discouraged with higher copayments.

Obviously, developing and maintaining a payment system of such complexity requires advanced information systems that can automate most processes and financial transactions. And consumers and patients will need an advocate who helps them understand their options and the consequences of their choices; the health navigator would fill this role.

Consumer Engagement

Consumers and patients will have to be engaged in their care decisions beyond cost-sharing. They need to be informed of their choices and the consequences of those choices: They are then free to select lifestyles, providers, and treatment options within the constraints of the PHM system. But while the PHM model as outlined in the previous chapters can offer them choices that promote better health and lower cost, actual engagement requires substantial patient education about disease, the role of self-management, and the effects and side effects of treatments so that patients can make truly informed decisions. More importantly, patients will need to progress from being passive recipients of medical advice to becoming experts in their own diseases and partners in care decisions. This ideal, set forth in the Chronic Care Model (Coleman et al., 2009), remains difficult to accomplish—especially in societies like that of China, which hold traditional views of the patient-physician relationship. But with better access to information and the support of the health navigator, Chinese citizens can move closer to becoming active and informed patients.

5.2. Care Delivery Under the Population Health Model

A health care system must address the health and medical needs of all of its citizens—particularly patients with chronic conditions that increasingly stretch existing infrastructure and resources. As Figure 5.2 shows, the health needs of a population and the goals of health care span a continuum from maintaining health and wellness, through recovering from acute illness and managing chronic conditions to coping with the end of life. Likewise, a health care delivery model must support the full continuum of health care. And each of these stages encompasses all dimensions of health, including physical, mental, and social well-being, as defined by the World Health Organi-

Figure 5.2
Health Needs and the Full Continuum of Health Care

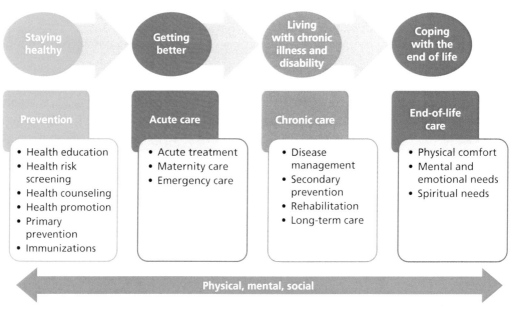

zation (Foundation for Accountability, 1997; Hurtado, Swift, and Corrigan, 2001; World Health Organization, 1948). Research has shown that managing health across the full continuum of care improves patient outcomes at relatively low cost (Mueller and MacKinney, 2006). In fact, the central tenet of the new ACO model in the United States is to manage care across the continuum, a goal that has remained elusive over the past five decades despite numerous attempts at reform (Rittenhouse, Shortell, and Fisher, 2009).

Health Promotion and Disease Prevention

Our analysis has shown that unhealthy lifestyles are an important contributor to the rising burden of chronic disease in China, as is typically the case in rapidly growing economies. Smoking rates are high, the traditionally healthy diet is being replaced by one laden with foods high in saturated fat and sugar, and physical activity is declining. To ensure the long-term health and productivity of the population, leaders need to implement a robust health promotion and disease prevention strategy that combines public health approaches—such as educational campaigns, taxes, and regulations—with personalized preventive services that would be delivered under the PHM.

The preventive services would include assessment of health behaviors (e.g., smoking status, diet, physical activity) and biometric screening (e.g., body-mass index, blood pressure, and lipid levels) followed by referrals to appropriate counseling and medical treatment services, when needed. To avoid overtaxing the medical care system, health promotion and disease prevention activities can leverage other existing institutions, such as public health agencies, school nurses, and workplace health staff. In particular, workplace health and wellness activities are now regarded as a preferred risk reduction strategy in Western countries, as employers have both access to and the trust of the adult population. A recent survey found that more than half of employers in the

Preventive Services Under the PHM—An Example

Mrs. Zhang is a 45-year-old woman who works as an administrative assistant for a local government agency. At the end of last year, she saw her primary care provider at the community health care center, within walking distance of her apartment complex, after her health navigator reminded her of an overdue preventive visit via emails and cell phone text messages. During her visit, her health navigator updated her personal health record with her current health behaviors (e.g., physical activity, diet, and smoking). Her physician did a physical exam and told her that she was healthy but needed to lose weight. At the end of the visit, a nutrition counselor met with with Mrs. Zhang and discussed the importance of weight control; recommended dietary changes, like avoiding fast food chains; and suggested she follow up with the team regarding the weight-control program.

United States offer wellness services, and most believe that they improve productivity and reduce health-related absences (Mattke et al., 2013).

Acute Care

Undoubtedly, China has made enormous progress in providing care for acute medical problems. Infant mortality rates have been falling and life expectancy at birth has been increasing continuously over the last half-century. Large cities have erected world-class hospitals, like the TEDA International Cardiovascular Hospital. Any future care delivery model needs to build upon this progress and incorporate current best practices to avoid overinvestment in redundant infrastructure:

- **Centers of excellence.** Hospitals that perform a high volume of complex procedures (e.g., cardiac surgery, pancreatectomy) are increasingly shown to achieve better outcomes (Halm, Lee, and Chassin, 2002; Markar et al., 2012; Soljak, 2002). Thus, provision of such services should be regionalized to a limited number of large academic medical centers.
- **Referral networks.** To allow centers of excellence to concentrate on their role, routine procedures need to be shifted to affiliated community hospitals. Rotation of staff through the network allows a large number of providers to be trained at the best centers and patients to see specialists close to their homes.
- **Deinstitutionalization.** Substantial evidence suggests that minimizing institutional (in-patient) care reduces cost and improves outcomes. Thus, the hospital of the future should perform many more procedures in the ambulatory setting

Acute Medical Services Under PHM—An Example

Mr. Li is a 24-year-old worker in a furniture factory. Three years ago, he was feeling unusually tired and called his health navigator for advice. The health navigator scheduled an appointment at the factory's clinic for the next morning. The clinic nurse took his vital signs, drew blood, and conducted a physical exam, which revealed that Mr. Li's right testicle was swollen. The nurse initiated a teleconsultation with a urologist in the community clinic who recommended blood tests, x-rays, a CT scan, and a testicular ultrasound. The health navigator scheduled the tests and a follow-up visit with the urologist two days later. The urologist confirmed to Mr. Li that he had a stage 4 seminoma but had an excellent prognosis. The urologist had already instructed the health navigator to book a bed at the city's main university hospital's cancer care center for surgery, radiation, and chemotherapy, and to inform Mr. Li's employer of the need for a prolonged medical leave. After two months of intensive therapy, Mr. Li was discharged home in full remission and made a quick recovery. He continues to do well, and his health navigator calls him regularly to schedule the recommended follow-up tests and visits.

and focus increasingly on hospital-to-home concepts (Shepperd and Iliffe, 2008; Shepperd et al., 2013). Providing care in patients' homes clearly reduces cost and allows them to recover in a familiar environment without the risk of hospital-acquired complications such as infections and confusion. At the same time, early discharge requires use of advanced remote monitoring technology and care coordination procedures to ensure a safe recovery.

Chronic Care

Our findings, particularly regarding the high mortality rate from NCDs, suggest that China needs to strengthen its infrastructure for chronic care delivery. While a robust prevention strategy, as we already outlined, will reduce the burden of chronic disease in the long run, its effects will take decades to materialize and will be undermined by the rapid aging of the population. A recent concept paper that RAND prepared for the World Health Organization argued that a successful strategy to reduce the burden of chronic disease must optimize the combination of prevention and treatment services for the local conditions (Mattke and Chow, 2012).

Western countries' lack of progress in improving chronic care delivery, in spite of high levels of spending, offers numerous lessons for China. In particular, China should focus on providing ongoing support, monitoring, and care management to avoid the limitations of an encounter-based medical system, and utilize patient-centered and team-based care, as we describe later. Traditional Chinese medicine should play an important role in providing symptom relief and health maintenance without incurring significant side effects.

Chronic Care Services Under PHM—An Example

Mrs. Wang is a 58-year-old merchandise manager of a retail chain and lives in a suburban area. Mrs. Wang was diagnosed with diabetes and hypertension three years ago during a routine exam at the community health center. Despite medical treatment, her physician could not get her blood pressure and glucose under sufficient control and referred her to an endocrinologist for consultation, who gave Mrs. Wang wireless glucose and blood pressure monitors and an electronic diabetes diary that would transmit data directly into her personal health record. After two months of data collection, the endocrinologist determined that Mrs. Wang had trouble adhering to her diet and medication regimen because of her busy travel schedule. The doctor adjusted Mrs. Wang's medication and referred her to a diabetes educator, who developed a personalized diabetes control program and recommended acupuncture for stress relief. Six months later, Mrs. Wang has learned how to maintain a healthy lifestyle even during extended travel and has gotten her blood pressure and glucose under control. Her health navigator reminds her regularly to visit the center for check-ups.

End-of-Life Care

Caring for terminally ill patients is a complex challenge that requires ensuring both physical comfort and culturally appropriate emotional and spiritual support (Foley and Gelband, 2013). Substantial data show that evidence-based palliative care improves patient comfort and reduces the use of futile medical interventions (Lorenz et al., 2008), but physicians are often reluctant to discuss this subject with patients and family members. This reluctance is particularly common in China, where family members strongly resist informing patients about their prognosis (Wang et al., 2004). With NCDs now accounting for the lion's share of mortality, China needs to develop culturally appropriate end-of-life care guidelines, train a pool of qualified professionals, and increase access to hospice care to avoid unnecessary hospital admissions for terminally ill patients.

CHAPTER SIX

Conclusions

China's economic and social progress over the past 50 years has outpaced the development of its health care system. The health of China's population is being influenced simultaneously by its rapid rate of aging, growing wealth, and migration from rural to urban living, as well as by greater reliance on food of low nutritional value and decreased physical activity. The result is an expanding burden of chronic disease and disability, even as mortality due to acute illness wanes. To handle the new challenge, the Chinese health care system must undergo a transformation.

The current system is handicapped by a severe workforce shortage (especially of nurses), overreliance on hospital-based care, and lack of robust IT. While the central government is investing substantial resources, the limited absorptive capacity of the current system makes it difficult to expand capacity fast enough to meet expected demand, at least with traditional delivery models. But China has the unique opportunity to chart a different course: Its relative freedom from legacy infrastructure and entrenched interests means it can adapt an innovative model for health care delivery that is purposefully designed for the 21st century, rather than emulating inefficient models that exist elsewhere.

This pioneering PHM model will be centered on the needs of citizens and offer continuous support at all stages of health. It will make use of sophisticated IT to leverage scarce medical professionals, improve quality, promote evidence-based care and accountability, and facilitate planning. It will become a source of service-sector jobs—not just in care delivery and management, but also in IT—and will help to promote economic growth by unlocking domestic savings. Thus, visionary leaders who embark on this ambitious agenda to transform health care in China can divert discontent about access to quality care as a threat to the harmonious society and use health care to promote the realization of the Chinese Dream.

References

Ahmad, K. (2000). South Korean doctors end crippling strike. *Lancet, 356*(9223), 54.

Arah, O. A., Westert, G. P., Hurst, J., and Klazinga, N. S. (2006). A conceptual framework for the OECD Health Care Quality Indicators Project. *International Journal for Quality in Health Care, 18 Suppl 1,* 5–13.

Barnett, S., Myrvoda, A., and Nabar, M. (2012, September). *Sino-spending.* International Monetary Fund website. Date accessed: June 24, 2013. Retrieved from: http://www.imf.org/external/pubs/ft/fandd/2012/09/barnett.htm

Berthold, H. K., Bestehorn, K. P., Jannowitz, C., Krone, W., and Gouni-Berthold, I. (2011). Disease management programs in type 2 diabetes: Quality of care. *American Journal of Managed Care, 17*(6), 393–403.

Berwick, D. M. (2011). Launching Accountable care organizations—The proposed rule for the Medicare Shared Savings Program. *New England Journal of Medicine, 364*(16), e32.

Berwick, D. M., Nolan, T. W., and Whittington, J. (2008). The triple aim: Care, health, and cost. *Health Affairs, 27*(3), 759–769.

Blumel, M., and Busse, R. (2009). Disease management programs—Time to evaluate. *Health Policy Monitor.*

Bodenheimer, T., Chen, E., and Bennett, H. D. (2009). Confronting the growing burden of chronic disease: Can the US health care workforce do the job? *Health Affairs, 28*(1), 64–74.

Brook, R. H. (1995). *The RAND/UCLA appropriateness method.* Santa Monica, CA: RAND Corporation, RP-395. Date accessed: June 24, 2013. Retrieved March 1, 2014 from: http://www.rand.org/pubs/reprints/RP395.html

Brooks, R., and Barnett, S. (2010). *China: Does government health and education spending boost consumption?* International Monetary Fund.

Burnside, C., and Dollar, D. (2004). Aid, policies, and growth: revisiting the evidence. World Bank Policy Research Working Paper (3251).

Busse, R. (2004). Disease management programs in Germany's statutory health insurance system. *Health Aff (Millwood), 23*(3), 56–67.

Busse, R., Nimptsch, U., and Mansky, T. (2009). Measuring, monitoring, and managing quality in Germany's hospitals. *Health Aff (Millwood), 28*(2), w294–w304.

Cabana, M. D., Rand, C. S., Powe, N. R., Wu, A. W., Wilson, M. H., Abboud, P. A., and Rubin, H. R. (1999). Why don't physicians follow clinical practice guidelines? A framework for improvement. *Journal of the American Medical Association, 282*(15), 1458–1465.

Centers for Disease Control and Prevention. (2012). *Lack of health insurance and type of coverage: Early release of selected estimates based on data from the 2011 National Health Interview Survey.*

———. (2013). *Faststats: diet/nutrition data for the U.S.* Date accessed: June 24, 2013. Retrieved from:
 http://www.cdc.gov/nchs/fastats/diet.htm

Centers for Sustainable Health Spending. (2013, April 10). *Health sector economic indicators; Insights from the Bureau of Labor Statistics (BLS) March 2013 employment data.* Altarium Institute.

Centers for Medicare and Medicaid Services. (2013). *Pioneer Accountable Care Organizations succeed in improving care, lowering costs.* Date accessed: June 24, 2013. Retrieved from:
https://www.cms.gov/Newsroom/MediaReleaseDatabase/Press-Releases/2013-Press-Releases-Items/2013-07-16.html

Chamon, M., and Prasad, E. (2008). *Why are saving rates of urban households in China rising?* National Bureau of Economic Research.

Charlton, R. (2005). Implications of the new GP contract. *Clinical Medicine, 5*(1), 50–54.

Chen, M. A., Hollenberg, J. P., Michelen, W., and Casalino, L. P. (2011). Patient care outside of office visits: A primary care physician time study. *Journal of General Internal Medicine, 26*(1), 58–63.

Cockcroft, L. (2007, October 31). Average salary for a GP leaps to £110,000, *Telegraph.* Date accessed: June 24, 2013. Retrieved from:
http://www.telegraph.co.uk/news/uknews/1567887/Average-salary-for-a-GP-leaps-to-110000.html

Coleman, K., Austin, B. T., Brach, C., and Wagner, E. H. (2009). Evidence on the Chronic Care Model in the new millennium. *Health Aff (Millwood), 28*(1), 75–85.

Coulter, A. (1999). Paternalism or partnership? Patients have grown up—and there's no going back. *BMJ, 319*(7212), 719–720.

Cristadoro, Riccardo, and Marconi, Daniela. (2012). Household savings in China. *Journal of Chinese Economic and Business Studies, 10*(3), 275–299.

Darmouth Institute for Health Policy and Clinical Practice. (2012). *The Dartmouth Atlas.* Date accessed: June 24, 2013. Retrieved from:
http://tdi.dartmouth.edu/about/contact-us

De Renzio, Paolo. (2009). Scaling up versus absorptive capacity: challenges and opportunities for reaching the MDGs in Africa. London: Overseas Development Institute.

Doctors' protest hobbles health care. (2000, February 18). *Los Angeles Times.* Date accessed: June 24, 2013. Retrieved from:
 http://articles.latimes.com/2000/feb/18/news/mn-253

Doran, T., Fullwood, C., Gravelle, H., Reeves, D., Kontopantelis, E., Hiroeh, U., and Roland, M. (2006). Pay-for-performance programs in family practices in the United Kingdom. *New England Journal of Medicine, 355*(4), 375–384.

Eaton, J., and Pell, M. (2011). *Lobbyists swarm Capitol to influence health reform.* The Center of Public Integrity. Date accessed: June 24, 2013. Retrieved from:
http://www.publicintegrity.org/2010/02/24/2725/lobbyists-swarm-capitol-influence-health-reform

Eggleston, K. (2012). *Health Care for 1.3 Billion: An Overview of China's Health System.* Stanford, CT.

Fang, X., Wang, X., and Bai, C. (2011). COPD in China; The burden and importance of proper management. *CHEST Journal, 139*(4), 920–929.

Fields, D., Leshen, E., and Patel, K. (2010). Analysis and commentary. Driving quality gains and cost savings through adoption of medical homes. *Health Aff (Millwood), 29*(5), 819–826.

Fisher, Elliott. (2013). Shift to Accountable Care Organizations. *The Wall Street Journal.* Date accessed: July 30, 2013. Retrieved from: http://blogs.wsj.com/experts/2013/07/19/elliott-fisher-shift-to-accountable-care-organizations/

Foley, K. M., and Gelband, H. (Eds.). (2013). *Improving Palliative Care for Cancer.* Washington, D.C. : National Academy Press.

Foundation for Accountability. (1997). Reporting quality information to consumers. Portland, Oregon: FACCT.

Gillam, S. J. (2011). *Pay for performance in UK General Practice–The ambiguous impact of the Quality and Outcomes Framework.* Agency for Healthcare Research and Quality. Date accessed: June 24, 2013. Retrieved from: http://www.qualitymeasures.ahrq.gov/expert/expert-commentary.aspx?id=25658

Halm, E. A., Lee, C., and Chassin, M. R. (2002). Is volume related to outcome in health care? A systematic review and methodologic critique of the literature. *Ann Intern Med,* 137(6), 511–520.

Hanson, K., Ranson, M. K., Oliveira-Cruz, V., and Mills, A. (2003). Expanding access to priority health interventions: A framework for understanding the constraints to scaling up. *Journal of International Development, 15*(1), 1–14.

Hibbard, J. H., and Greene, J. (2013). What the evidence shows about patient activation: Better health outcomes and care experiences; fewer data on costs. *Health Aff (Millwood), 32*(2), 207–214.

Hillestad, R., Bigelow, J., Bower, A., Girosi, F., Meili, R., Scoville, R., and Taylor, R. (2005). Can electronic medical record systems transform health care? Potential health benefits, savings, and costs. *Health Aff (Millwood), 24*(5), 1103–1117.

Hu, J. (2012). *Keynote Address.* Paper presented at the 18th CPC National Congress, Great Hall of the People, Beijing.

Hurtado, M. P., Swift, E. K., and Corrigan, J. M. (2001). *Envisioning the national health care quality report.* Washington, DC: National Academies Press.

IMS Institute for Healthcare Informatics. (2013). *Avoidable costs in U.S. healthcare: The $200 billion opportunity from using medicines more responsibly.* Date accessed: June 24, 2013. Retrieved from: http://www.imshealth.com/deployedfiles/imshealth/Global/Content/Corporate/IMS%20Institute/RUOM-2013/IHII_Responsible_Use_Medicines_2013.pdf

Institute of Medicine. (1999). *To err is human: Building a safer health system.* Washington, D.C.: National Academy of Sciences.

Institute of Medicine. (2011). *Clinical practice guidelines we can trust.* Washington, D.C.: National Academy of Sciences.

Institute of Medicine Committee on Quality of Health Care in America. (2001). *Crossing the quality chasm: A new health system for the 21st century.* Washington, DC: National Academies Press.

Jha, A. K., Doolan, D., Grandt, D., Scott, T., and Bates, D. W. (2008). The use of health information technology in seven nations. *Int J Med Inform, 77*(12), 848–854.

Kaiser Family Foundation. (2013). *Health expenditure per capita (PPP; international $).* Date accessed: June 24, 2013. Retrieved from: http://kff.org/global-indicator/health-expenditure-per-capita/

Kellermann, A. L., and Jones, S. S. (2013). What it will take to achieve the as-yet-unfulfilled promises of health information technology. *Health Aff (Millwood), 32*(1), 63–68.

Kim, H., and Ruger, J. P. (2008). Pharmaceutical reform in South Korea and the lessons it provides. *Health Affairs, 27*(4), w260–w269.

Lee, Kheng Hock. (2008). The hospitalist movement—a complex adaptive response to fragmentation of care in hospitals. *Annals—Academy of Medicine Singapore, 37*(2), 145.

Lester, H., Sharp, D. J., Hobbs, F. D. R., and Lakhani, M. (2006). The quality and outcomes framework of the GMS contract: A quiet evolution for 2006. *The British Journal of General Practice, 56*(525), 244.

Liberto, J. (2011). Health care lobbying boom continues. CNN.com. Date accessed: June 24, 2013. Retrieved from:
http://money.cnn.com/2011/03/25/news/economy/health_care_lobbying/index.htm

Liu, X. (2013, May 19). Service industry's contribution to economic growth surpassed manufacturing for the first time in the first quarter of 2013, *People's Daily*. Date accessed: June 24, 2013. Retrieved from:
http://paper.people.com.cn/rmrb/html/2013-05/19/nw.D110000renmrb_20130519_1-01.htm

Liu, Y., Rao, K., Wu, J., and Gakidou, E. (2008). China's health system performance. *The Lancet, 372*(9653), 1914–1923.

Lorenz, K. A., Lynn, J., Dy, S. M., Shugarman, L. R., Wilkinson, A., Mularski, R. A., et al. (2008). Evidence for improving palliative care at the end of life: a systematic review. *Ann Intern Med, 148*(2), 147–159.

Markar, S. R., Karthikesalingam, A., Thrumurthy, S., and Low, D. E. (2012). Volume-outcome relationship in surgery for esophageal malignancy:Systematic review and meta-analysis 2000–2011. *Journal of Gastrointestinal Surgery, 16*(5), 1055–1063.

Mattke, S. (2004). Monitoring and improving the technical quality of medical care: A new challenge for policymakers in OECD countries. In The OECD Health Project (Eds.), *Towards high-performing health systems.* Paris: OECD Publications.

Mattke, S., and Chow, J. C. (2012). *Measuring health system progress in reducing mortality from noncommunicable diseases.* Santa Monica, CA: RAND Corporation, OP-380-HLTH. Date accessed: March 1, 2014. Retrieved from:
http://www.rand.org/pubs/occasional_papers/OP380.html

Mattke, S., Liu, H., Caloyeras, J. P., Huang, C. Y., Van Busum, K. R., Khodyakov, D., and Shier, V. (2013). *Workplace Wellness Programs Study.* Santa Monica, CA: RAND Corporation, RR-254-DOL. Accessed: March 1, 2014. Retrieved from:
http://www.rand.org/pubs/research_reports/RR254.html

Meng, Q., and Tang, S. (2010). Universal coverage of health care in China: Challenges and opportunities. *World Health Report.*

Miksch, A., Laux, G., Ose, D., Joos, S., Campbell, S., Riens, B., and Szecsenyi, J. (2010). Is there a survival benefit within a German primary care-based disease management program? *American Journal of Managed Care, 16*(1), 49–54.

Mueller, K. J., and MacKinney, A. C. (2006). Care across the continuum: Access to health care services in rural America. *The Journal of Rural Health, 22*(1), 43–49.

Myanmar Phar-med Expo 2013. (2013). News; Government suspends plan to build 4 hospitals in the capital. Date accessed: June 24, 2013. Retrieved from:
http://pharmed-myanmar.com/index.php/news/government-suspends-plan-to-build-4-hospitals-in-the-capital.html

National Bureau of Statistics of China. (2006). *China statistical yearbook.* Beijing, China: China Statistics Press.

———. (2007). *China statistical yearbook.* Beijing, China: China Statistics Press.

———. (2011). *China statistical yearbook.* Beijing, China: China Statistics Press.

———. (2012). *China statistical yearbook.* Beijing, China: China Statistics Press.

National eHealth Collaborative. (2010). *The Patient engagement framework.* Date accessed: June 24, 2013. Retrieved from:
http://www.nationalehealth.org/patient-engagement-framework

NHS Employers. (May 10, 2013). *Quality and outcomes framework.* Date accessed: June 24, 2013. Retrieved from:
http://www.nhsemployers.org/payandcontracts/generalmedicalservicescontract/qof/Pages/QualityOutcomesFramework.aspx

Nolte, E., Knai, C., Hofmarcher, M., Conklin, A., Erler, A., Elissen, A.,et al. (2012). Overcoming fragmentation in health care: Chronic care in Austria, Germany and the Netherlands. [Research Support, Non-U.S. Gov't Review]. *Health economics, policy, and law, 7*(1), 125–146.

Office of the National Coordinator for Health Information Technology. (2013). *Policymaking, regulation and strategy: Clinical decision support (CDS).* Date accessed: June 24, 2013. Retrieved from http://www.healthit.gov/policy-researchers-implementers/clinical-decision-support-cds

Organization for Economic Cooperation Development. (2011). *Health at a glance 2011: OECD indicators.* OECD.

———. (2012a). *Health at a glance 2012: OECD indicators.* OECD.

———. (2012b). *Health at a glance: Asia/Pacific 2012.* OECD.

Quadagno, J. (2011). Interest-Group Influence on the Patient Protection and Affordability Act of 2010: Winners and Losers in the Health Care Reform Debate. *Journal of Health Politics, Policy and Law, 36*(3), 449–453.

Rittenhouse, D. R., Shortell, S. M., and Fisher, E. S. (2009). Primary care and accountable care—two essential elements of delivery-system reform. *New England Journal of Medicine, 361*(24), 2301–2303.

Rosenthal, T. C. (2008). The medical home: Growing evidence to support a new approach to primary care. *J Am Board Fam Med, 21*(5), 427–440.

Scottish Government. (2011, December 18). *More-Scottish-focused GP contract.* Date accessed: June 24, 2013. Retrieved from:
http://www.scotland.gov.uk/News/Releases/2011/12/19102020

Shepperd, S., and Iliffe, S. (2008). Hospital at home versus in-patient hospital care (Review). In Cochrane Effective Practice and Organisation of Care Group (Ed.), *The Cochrane collaboration.* The Cochrane Library.

Shepperd, S., Lannin, N. A., Clemson, L. M., McCluskey, A., Cameron, I. D., and Barras, S. L. (2013). Discharge planning from hospital to home (Review). In Cochrane Effective Practice and Organisation of Care Group (Ed.), *The Cochrane collaboration.* The Cochrane Library.

Skocpol, T. (1997). *Boomerang: Health care reform and the turn against government.* WW Norton and Company.

Smith, P. C., and York, N. (2004). Quality incentives: the case of UK general practitioners. *Health Affairs, 23*(3), 112–118.

Soljak, M. (2002). Volume of procedures and outcome of treatment. *BMJ, 325*(7368), 787–788.

Steinbrook, R. (2009). Lobbying, campaign contributions, and health care reform. *New England Journal of Medicine, 361*(23).

Szecsenyi, J., Rosemann, T., and Joos, S. (2008). German diabetes disease management programs are appropriate for restructuring care according to the chronic care model. *Diabetes Care, 31*(6).

Stoto, M. A. (2013). Population health in the Affordable Care Act era. *AcademyHealth.* Date accessed: June 24, 2013. Retrieved from: http://www.academyhealth.org/files/AH2013pophealth.pdf

Tanner, M. S. (2005). *Chinese government responses to rising social unrest.* Santa Monica, CA: RAND Corporation, CT-240. Date accessed: June 24, 2013. Retrieved from: http://www.rand.org/pubs/testimonies/CT240.html

Timbie, J. W., Fox, D. S., Van Busum, K., and Schneider, E. C. (2012). Five reasons that many comparative effectiveness studies fail to change patient care and clinical practice. *Health Affairs, 31*(10), 2168–2175.

Tuck, M. (April, 2013). *Poverty.* Date accessed: June 24, 2013. Retrieved from: http://go.worldbank.org/VL7N3V6F20

U.S. Congress, Office of Technology Assessment. (1995). *Hospital financing in seven countries.* Washington, DC.

United Nations. (2012). *World population prospects, the 2012 revision.* Date accessed: June 24, 2013. Retrieved from: http://esa.un.org/wpp/Excel-Data/population.htm

Wang, S., Marquez, M., and Langenbrunner, J. (2011). Toward a healthy and harmonious life in China: Stemming the rising tide of noncommunicable diseases. *Human Development Unit.*

Wang, X. S., Di, L. J., Reyes-Gibby, C. C., Guo, H., Liu, S. J., and Cleeland, C. S. (2004). End-of-life care in urban areas of China: A survey of 60 oncology clinicians. *J Pain Symptom Manage, 27*(2), 125–132.

Watts, Jonathan. (2001). Korea's pharmacists protest against drug law reforms. *The Lancet, 357*(9257), 697.

What can be learned from China's health system? (2012). *The Lancet, 379*(9818), 777.

World Bank. (undated-a). *GDP growth (annual %).* Date accessed: June 24, 2013. Retrieved from:

http://data.worldbank.org/indicator/NY.GDP.MKTP.KD.ZG/

————. (undated-b). *Life expectancy at birth, total (years).* Date accessed: June 24, 2013. Retrieved from: http://data.worldbank.org/indicator/SP.DYN.LE00.IN

World Health Organization. (1948). *WHO definition of health.* Date accessed: June 24, 2013. Retrieved from: http://www.who.int/about/definition/en/print.html

————. (2005). *Facing the facts: The impact of chronic disease in China.* Date accessed: June 24, 2013. Retrieved from: http://www.who.int/chp/chronic_disease_report/media/china.pdf

————. (2011). *NCD country profiles: China.* Date accessed: June 24, 2013. Retrieved from:

http://www.who.int/nmh/countries/chn_en.pdf?ua=1

———. (2013). *Mortality: All NCDs, deaths per 100,000 by country.* Date accessed: June 24, 2013. Retrieved from:
http://apps.who.int/gho/data/node.main.A863?lang=en

World Health Organization Global Health Observatory. (2008). *Noncommunicable diseases: Risk factors.* Date accessed: June 24, 2013. Retrieved from:
http://apps.who.int/gho/data/node.main.A867?lang=en

Yescombe, E. R. (2011). *Public-private partnerships: Principles of policy and finance:* Butterworth-Heinemann.

Yip, W. C., Hsiao, W. C., Chen, W., Hu, S., Ma, J., and Maynard, A. (2012). Early appraisal of China's huge and complex health-care reforms. *The Lancet, 379*(9818), 833–842.

Yip, W. C., Hsiao, W., Meng, Q., Chen, W., and Sun, X. (2010). Realignment of incentives for health-care providers in China. *The Lancet, 375*(9720), 1120–1130.

Yip, W., and Hsiao, W. C. (2008). The Chinese health system at a crossroads. *Health Affairs, 27*(2), 460–468.

Zhang, Y., Xu, Y., Nie, H., Lei, T., Wu, Y., Zhang, L., and Zhang, M. (2012). Prevalence of dementia and major dementia subtypes in the Chinese populations: A meta-analysis of dementia prevalence surveys, 1980–2010. *Journal of Clinical Neuroscience, 19*(10), 1333–1337.

Zhao, J., Zhang, Z., Guo, H., Li, Y., Xue, W., Ren, L., et al. (2010). E-health in China: Challenges, initial directions, and experience. *Telemedicine and e-Health, 16*(3), 344–349.